I0468244

What's going on in your gut?

The complete guide to Probiotics and the health benefits
they offer

MARTIN MEYER

Legal & Disclaimer

Legal & Disclaimer

The information contained in this book is not designed to replace or take the place of any form of medicine or professional medical advice. The information in this book has been provided for educational and entertainment purposes only.

The information contained in this book has been compiled from sources deemed reliable, and it is accurate to the best of the Author's knowledge; however, the Author cannot guarantee its accuracy and validity and cannot be held liable for any errors or omissions. Changes are periodically made to this book. You must consult your doctor or get professional medical advice before using any of the suggested remedies, techniques, or information in this book.

Upon using the information contained in this book, you agree to hold harmless the Author from and against any damages, costs, and expenses, including any legal fees potentially resulting from the application of any of the information provided by this guide. This disclaimer applies to any damages or injury caused by the use and application, whether directly or indirectly, of any advice or information presented,

Table of Contents

Introduction

I am betting that you like most of the population have never taken the time to read an end user license agreement, just opting to tick the box at the end. Sound familiar? Whilst you may not physically read the agreement what about the rest of you? The trillions of microscopic creatures that live in your eyes, ears and within your stomach that make up the world within your body that offers the potential to redefine how you understand disease, your health and you!

Thanks to the ever growing technology, scientists today know far more about the microscopic life forms that reside inside you that ever before, and what the findings reveal is quite astonishing. The single celled microbes are not only more numerous that you could ever imagine but they live in nearly every area of your body and are far more important and play a role in every aspect of your health.

This collection of microscopic creatures that have set up home on and within you are more commonly referred to as human microbiota, and their genes are known as the human microbiome. Charting this human microbiome has taught us that even our own bodies are complete with a mass of independent and interdependent life forms that have their own specific goals and agendas.

The human body is made up of approximately 10 trillion human cells and there are about 100 trillion microbial cells in and on your body. We are not as previously thought just an unlucky host to the occasional bad bug that gives us an infection. The fact is that we live in balance with an entire community of microbes, and they are not just passengers, these tiny organisms play essential roles in the most basic processes in our lives including our immune responses, digestion and even our behavior.

This inner group of microbes is actually a number of different groups with different sets of microbes living within the different parts of the body where they play specific roles. The microbes that live in the mouth are completely different from those that are living on your skin or in your stomach. Have you ever thought why some people are tastier to mosquitoes than others? It is true that some people are far more appetizing! The important reasoning for this is the different groups of microbes on the skin, and it doesn't end there, as there is an extraordinary variety of microbes that live in and on each one of us. You probably know that we are all very similar with regards to our human DNA, in terms of our human DNA we are 99.99% identical to the person who you are sitting next too, however this is not true when it comes to your gut microbes, you may share just 10%. It is these differences that account for the huge variations between humans such as weight to allergies and the likelihood of getting sick to anxiety levels. It is true that we have only just begun to understand the vast microscopic world but the implications of these findings are amazing.

The unbelievable assortment of the microbial world is even more intriguing as until 40 years ago we were unaware of how many singe celled organisms there are or the many variations. Until this time all our ideas on the worlds living things came from Charles Darwin. Darwin produced a progressive tree which grouped all living things together by their shared physical traits. This traditional picture of life was based entirely on what people could see around them or through microscopes, the larger living things were classified as animals, plants and fungi; however the picture of the single celled organisms was completely wrong.

Carl Woese and George E Fox the American microbiologists in 1977 mapped a tree of life by comparing life forms at cellular level using a relative of DNA known as ribosomnal RNA that is found in every cell and used to make proteins. The results were astounding as it revealed single celled organisms to be far more diverse than all plants and animals combined. It turns out that animals, plants, fungi, humans etc in fact in all life we can see three short twigs that come from one branch of the tree of life and it is the single celled organisms, bacteria, archaea, yeasts and others that dominate.

In the past few years we have made amazing advancements in our understanding of microscopic life within us. Improvements in DNA sequencing combined with the explosion of computer power has been the key, and now through a process known as next generation sequencing we are capable of collecting cell samples from various parts of the body in order to identify the microbial DNA that they contain and combine the information from samples across the body to identify the thousands of different microbes that live on us. We are uncovering bacteria, archaea, yeasts and other single celled organisms that have their own genetics to define them all of the time.

New computer algorithms are making it far easier to interpret all of this genetic information. It is possible for us to now create a map of our microbes in order to compare the varieties in the different areas of our body and compare how different varieties are in one person to another. The majority of this new information comes from a $170 million research called the Human Microbiome Project which is sponsored by the US National Institutes of Health. Through this project more than 200 scientists have analyzed vast DNA and this is just the start.

The cost of all of this analysis is dropping rapidly meaning that more people are able to obtain a complete statement of the life within them. Just 10 years ago if you had wanted to know your microbiome make up it would have cost you $100 million, yet today exactly the same information will cost just $100! It is for this reason that it has been suggested this may soon be a routine test ordered by your doctor. Why though would your doctor want to know about your microbiome? The answer is simple and it is because new research is emerging that indicate previously unknown links between our microbes and a number of diseases which include autism, depression, arthritis and obesity and as these links become more apparent so are glimmers of future treatments.

Nearly everything that you can possibly imagine has an effect on the microbiome, such as diet, medicine, whether you are the oldest child or even the number of sexual partners you have had.

You will discover as you read through this book we are continually discovering that microbes are deeply integrated into nearly every aspect of our lives, in fact microbes are redefining exactly what it means to be human.

This book has been written to cover the following topics in depth and provide you with a full understand of Probiotics and how they can assist you to a happier and healthier life.

- The microscopic life that lives within you
- Where does microbiome come from?
- In sickness and health
- How microbes affect your mind, mood and more
- Probiotics and how to build yourself better microbiome
- The future of human microbiome

Chapter 1 – The microscopic life that lives within you

If you were to go by weight the average adult has about 3 pounds of microbes living inside of them. This means that the microbiome is one of the largest organs in the body, about the weight of your brain and slightly lighter than your liver.

From the introduction we can deduce in terms of sheer volume of cells, the microbial cells in our bodies outnumber the human cells by up to one in every ten, and of we were to measure by DNA, each person has about 20,000 microbial genes, therefore genetically speaking we are all at least 99% microbe!

The organisms which live within and on us are varied and there are copious amounts of them, with the majority being single celled organisms. It is possible that you could find members of the archaea which are single celled organisms that have no nuclei with the most common being the methanogens which are creatures that exist without oxygen, help to digest our food and excrete methane gas. There are also the eukaryotes such as the fungi of athlete's foot and the yeasts that grow in the vagina and occasionally our gut. The most dominant of all our bacteria such as Escherichia coli, originally thought of as an illness caught from under washed spinach, actually lives in harmless and helpful versions within most human intestines.

With the help of new technology a new discovery is made daily regarding the diversity of these creatures and many more are realized. For example, you may think that any two bacteria in your stomach feeding on the same source are pretty similar, when actually there are two bacteria with completely different behaviors, ecological roles and nutritional sources.

<u>Where are our microbes and what do they do?</u>

The easiest way for us to see where our microbes are and what they do is to look at the various parts of the body. Scientists are still trying to work out the productive purposes of the creatures that live on our largest organ the skin, but they have confirmed that these creatures contribute to our body odor. These microbes metabolize the chemicals that the skin produces into various volatile organic compounds, which bugs like or dislike.

Anopheles gambiae is one of the main species of mosquitoes which transmit malaria, and it picks up on the alluring odor that is surprisingly not coming from our armpits but actually from our hands and feet. This raises the question of whether rubbing antibiotics into the hands and feet would ward off an attack of this species as by killing the microbes you are actually killing the smell.

Like all of our microbes, the ones on our skin do not necessarily exist for our benefit; however as benign inhabitants they help us immensely by residing upon us making it harder for nasty microbes to infect us. Different areas of the skin have different microbes on then and the diversity and number is not necessarily linked to the number of individual microbes you have in a particular area.

Your armpits and forehead have many microbes but few species whereas the palm of the hand and forearm are sparse microbial habitats, but many species accumulate there. Women appear to have more varied microbial communities on their hands than men, and these differences survive hand washing suggesting that they could come from biological differences however the cause is still unknown.

Studies have shown that microbes which live on your left hand are different from those residing on the right. Even though our hands are touching the same surfaces each develop distinct microbial communities. It is this that inspired a professor of ecology and evolutionary biology at the University of Colorado and others to try and reproduce one of the famous findings in biology. The professor developed a very elaborate theory of biogeography to try and explain the dispersal of organisms among islands, and the relationship between the variety of species and the area that they populate. There was a split discovered that runs through Malaysia and Indonesia which separate the Asian fauna from the Australian fauna. The research went further by looking at the letters G & H on a computer with distinct populations from the users left and right hands being seen, and tests being undertaken from the space bar to see whether this had more type of microbes because it is larger than the other keys.

These studies showed some remarkable results and this was that each fingertip and its corresponding key had the same microbial groups. It was possible to match up a computer mouse with over 90% certainty to the palm of the hand of the user. This could be due to the microbes on the hands being very distinctive in one person to another with an average of 85% of the various species proving that humans also have a microbial fingerprint.

Research has progressed further with experiments to understand how many times you would need to touch an object in order to leave detectable microbial traces; however the results are still too questionable to be used.

<u>Nose and lungs</u>

Moving on to the nose it has been proved that the human nostril is home to its own specific and distinctive microbes which include staphylococcus aureus the bacteria that causes staph infections in hospitals. Healthy people it seems are often home to dangerous microbes and it is believed that other bacteria in the nose can prevent the staphylococcus aureus to take hold. It has also been shown that the environment has great influence on the types of microbes that gather in our noses. Children who have more varied types of bacteria in their noses for example those that live on or near farms are far less likely to develop asthma and allergies as they grow up. In other words playing in the dirt can actually be good for you!

When it comes to our lungs we only usually find dead bacteria. The air exposed surfaces of the lungs contain a mixture of antimicrobial peptides which are tiny proteins that kill the bacteria as soon as it lands. In people that are sick with cystic fibrosis or HIV harmful microbes can be found which contribute to pulmonary disease.

It is still not known whether the throat houses its own distinct microbes from the mouth passing through it. However it has been proven that the microbes in the throat of a smoker are different from a non smoker and this could show that smoking is not just harmful to the individual but also to some of the creatures that live within us.

Mouth and stomach

The chances are that you have only ever heard about bad bacteria in the mouth that cause gum disease and tooth decay. One of the bad bugs is streptococcus mutans, which like to eat teeth! This bug appears to have grown along with human agriculture which has made our diets richer in carbohydrates in particular sugars. Just as we have inadvertently made rats domesticated to eat food from our rubbish bins, bacterial vermin have become domesticated to live in our body. Luckily the majority of domesticated bacteria in our mouths is beneficial and form biofilms which keep out bad bacteria. The microbes in our mouth may even help to regulate our blood pressure by relaxing our arteries with a compound that helps to produce nitric oxide.

Fusobacterium nucleatum is usually found in healthy mouths but can also contribute to periodontal disease. Fusobacterium nucleatum is interesting as it has been seen within the tumors of those with colon cancer. It is not known whether this association is the cause or the effect. Fusobacterium nucleatum might produce the disease or it could be simply responding to the environment where the tumor lives. Even the different sides of the same tooth can harbor their own microbial groups, which may be influenced by a number of factors including oxygen exposure and chewing patterns.

Deep within the stomach is a highly acidic environment where only a few types of microbes can survive, however these microbes can be really important. Of particular note are Helicobacter pylori which have lived with us for so long it is impossible to know which humans are closely related and who they came into contact with as this bug grew. Helicobacter pylori play a vital role with regards to stomach ulcers which are sores in the stomach or small intestine where the protective mucus lining has worn away allowing the gastric acid to eat the body's tissue. The symptoms begin with bad breath and burning stomach pain which gains momentum and leads to nausea and bleeding from both ends. Previously doctors had blamed these ulcers on stress and diet advising that the individual relax, cut out spicy foods, coffee and alcohol and recommending antacids and milk, whilst patients had some relief they rarely recovered.

During the 80s a pair of Australian physicians proved that the majority of ulcers are caused by the Helicobacter pylori infections and they can be treated effectively with a course of antibiotics or the chemical bismuth which targets the bacteria. It has become apparent today that half of the human population carries Helicobacter pylori, with this in mind though why don't all people have ulcers? It transpires that Helicobacter pylori is just one of the many risk factors for ulcers, Helicobacter pylori appears to be something that many humans carry with no complaint.

Intestines

The intestines are believed to be the largest and most important microbial community in the body and if you are a microbe living on a human this is the main place to be! About 20 – 30 feet long, the intestine is fill of nooks and crannies making it the ideal place for microbes as it is warm and offers plenty to eat and drink as well as a convenient sewer system.

Most of the nutrients from your food are absorbed into the bloodstream by the small intestine and it is the large intestine that absorbs the water and the helpful microbes that ferment the fiber in the diet that passes undigested from the small intestine. These helpful microbes work alongside the digestive system making them the gatekeepers of our metabolism. The microbes have the potential to influence what we eat and how many calories we get as well as what nutrients and toxins we are exposed to and how drugs cab affect us all.

The other main fact about this highly important microbial community is that it is easy to obtain samples and although there are differences between the microbes found in the small and large intestines the variation is tiny when compared with those found within individual people. From this it can be deduced that your poo is a great way to understand and find out what microbes are unique to your gut. You should note though that the picture derived from your poo is really distorted. E coli has made the headlines as an ominous bacteria that on occasions makes its way into food, however it appears that this is not such a menacing bacteria when it is on its own. E coli are not a major player in the gut and make up just one cell in every ten thousand of most healthy adults.

The majority of bacteria found in the gut are far more fickle and it is not yet known how these can be grown in a lab, and the two main groups of bacteria are more often referred to as Bacteroidetes and Firmicutes, both of which are vital for digesting foods and metabolizing drugs. They have also been strongly linked to obesity, colon cancer, inflammatory bowel disease, multiple sclerosis, heart disease and autism. This is why techniques such as next generation DNA sequencing are such a revolution allowing us to look at what until now has been invisible.

Genitals

As of now very little is known about the microbes that live on and inside the penis, and whilst modern microbiology hasn't taken a really close look at this, some progress has been made. The vagina however has been studied extensively. In healthy adults of European ancestry the vagina is generally dominated by a few species of Lactobacillus. Although these are not the same species found in yoghurt they are very closely related and produce lactic acid which keeps the vagina acidic. The species that dominate a particular vagina can vary over time such as during the menstrual cycle when iron metabolizing bacteria Deferribacter feed on the blood. Vaginal bacteria can also change when a women starts sleeping with a new partner.

Until recently the majority of research undertaken on vaginal bacteria has been focused on sexually transmitted infections. There has been a lot of research into the role that vaginal microbes may help or hinder the transmission of various sexually transmitted diseases including HIV.

Research has proved that not all healthy vaginal microbes look similar to the extent that different populations have really different healthy families of vaginal microbes, and vaginal microbes do to the same extent define a women's destiny.

Chapter 2 – Where do microbiome come from?

All parents want the best for their children from conception all the way through their lives. Whilst it is apparent that a doctors job is to deliver children successfully with the intervention of modern medicine when necessary, however what may come as a surprise is that today's medical technology doesn't supply everything.

When it comes to the microbes of a newborn that has been born by cesarean section, it is down to parents to take matters into their own hands, and this is what those in the know have chosen to do. Generally what people fail to realize is babies born by cesarean are not getting the microbes that pass from mother to a newborn that has passed through the birth canal, and it is down to the parents to correct this. The process involves taking swabs from the mother's vagina and transferring to the skin, ears and mouth of the newborn.

The reason for these actions can be explained as follows, everyone gets their first microbes from their mother when they pass through the birth canal and there is evidence that before someone is even born their mother's microbiome is preparing for them. During pregnancy there is a particular kind of Lactobacillus that begin to dominate the vagina as the population in her gut starts to shift towards those more efficient at extracting the energy from what she eats. However this population unfortunately is more likely to cause inflammation of the gut particularly in the third trimester.

But how is it that we know the microbiome of a woman changes during pregnancy? This is thanks to a team of international scientists who transferred a stool from a pregnant lady to mice being raised in a sterile bubble, which meant they had no microbes of their own. The mice were then divided into two groups, one which received the fecal matter whilst the others received the same but from a woman in her third trimester. By the scientist transplanting these microbes into mice, it was possible to investigate whether the changes were as a response to pregnancy or merely just catalysts. The microbial communities in the guts of the pregnant women may be changing so the mother can extract more energy or nutrients from her diet to pass to her baby. It is also possible that those gut microbes are preparing to pass themselves onto the fetus, as this is what happens in animals with specialized diets for example koalas which need to digest eucalyptus leaves.

It is not clear whether we have microbes whilst in the uterus, there has been reports that link microbes in the amniotic fluid or placenta to preterm birth, however these initial findings have yet to be reproduced. Currently it is believed that a healthy fetus probably doesn't have any bacteria, although as with all research this information may be subject to change as new data accumulates.

Your first microbes probably come from birth and are gained by passing thought your mother's birth canal which is lined with vaginal bacteria. Whilst different women can have different vaginal microbial communities however during pregnancy their microbial communities all move into the same state. Assuming that a baby's first microbes come from the birth canal and vagina what happens to those not born this way? Birth by cesarean section is on the rise, either because of the rising rates of medical complications or maybe just because they are easier to schedule. Unlike adults, who have many distinctive microbial structures, the microbiomes in newborns appear very much the same. When delivered vaginally their microbes mirror that of their mother's vaginal communities, whilst those delivered by cesarean have microbes which are found on the mother's skin, and are a totally different community. Cesarean births have been linked to higher rates of various diseases that are associated with microbiome and or the immune system including asthma. Although there are conflicting studies currently this could also include obesity, atopic disease or skin rash and food allergies. Please do not be alarmed if your child was born by cesarean as the most likely outcome is that they will be fine, as this is a relatively small risk even though it makes perfect sense that missing exposure to a community of microbes may lead to health issues.

At the time of writing this book, scientists have confirmed that vaginal and cesarean babies have different microbiome at birth. As yet though there is not enough information to determine if or how this has an impact on health later in life. It is extremely difficult to determine the effects of cesarean versus vaginal birth as once we are born our microbiome becomes complex and whilst all those born through the birth canal have very similar microbiome by the time that they reach adulthood there are huge differences.

If we can be so different from one another, it makes perfect sense to wonder who we are similar too. Is it those who eat the same food as us? Is it the family that we share our home with? Is it the other people in our city or country? As it turns out all of these factors influence our microbiome and it has only recently come to light that some are more important than others.

The most profound period for the development of our microbes is whilst we are infants. Research was undertaken to study a boy from the first stool produced through his first 2 years and 3 months. The boy was delivered vaginally and the boy's gut microbiome showed he had an adult woman's vaginal community in his stool which is to be expected however eventually this develops into a normal looking adult microbiome however it is the time in the middle where there is so much variation. Day to day the differences in the child's stool communities are far larger than the differences between the fecal microbes of two healthy people.

Microbial speaking the boy starts off looking similar to a bear and ends up resembling a monkey. One thing that is apparent is when a child is taking antibiotics their microbiome makes him not only look like a different person but also like a different species. This in turn raises questions about how frequently we dose our children and ourselves with antibiotics.

Our diets help to shape our microbiome from very early on and there are substantial changes seen from breast feeding versus formula feeding. An infant that is breast fed is exposed to special microbes found in breast milk as well as special sugars which promote the growth of beneficial microbes. The child's microbiome evolves further when they start solid foods.

In the long term you are what you eat and your diet over a period of a year has one of the largest effects seen on gut microbiome adjusting the balance of two major groups of bacteria that digest dietary fiber and protein. These two categories of intestinal bacteria also account for gut microbiome and prove that along with distinct languages and cultures different people around the world also have distinctive gut microbes. Bacteroides found predominately in people who eat high meat diets whereas Prevotella are more abundant in the gut of those that eat a high grain diet.

You may wonder how diet manipulates your microbiome. To date very few studies have been carried out, however connections that have been discovered suggests there are pervasive effects between diet and malnutrition, infection risk and acne.

The environmental influence on the microbiome is profound in childhood, however this is not surprising when you consider your children, then stick their fingers in everything imaginable and then stick their filthy fingers straight in their mouth! It does transpire thought that this isn't all bad. Children that have more diverse microbial communities are those who have been exposed to a range of influences and as such have far lower immune system defects such as hay fever than those children who have grown up in cities.

The majority of things we do will not change our microbes that much because our microbiome remains distinctive even as they age. Later in life people tend to have diverse gut microbial communities overall. In one respect the last days of our lives resembles our first as E coli and its relatives tend to be common both in the elderly and infants. There is no definitive reason for this; it could be that they recognize the sick gut of the elderly and the undeveloped gut of the infant.

If it came down to it and you had to replace your microbiome, would you choose the microbes from a centenarian, a child or someone of your own age? It is possible that the centenarian have really healthy gut microbiome and this is how they have reached old age, however it could also be that despite their heroic service they are on their last legs and therefore transplanting them would not be advisable. In the same way, transplanting a youthful microbiome may appear to be a good way to obtain a young and vigorous community to develop, however suppose a microbe was beneficial at a young age but detrimental in advancing years. At this point there has been little research completed and science cannot at this time help.

Chapter 3 – In sickness and health

Scientists are continually amazed by discoveries that link the power that the microbiome has with regards to shaping and defining what we become. What is most exciting is the real prospect that as we get a better understanding and are able to influence the microbiome, it may give us the power to heal ourselves.

It is already possible to link our microbes to a wide variety of specific diseases, from the obvious infectious ones and inflammatory bowel disease to some surprising ones such as multiple sclerosis, depression and autism. It should be noted that although we know that a certain microbe is involved in a specific disease it doesn't mean that the cure is to eliminate that microbe, as doing so may actually cause irreversible damage. It may be that targeting diet or inhibiting enzymes may be more effective than attacking the microbes directly. The reason there is such excitement about the microbiome is the possibility that it could help to uncover completely new mechanisms that can treat conditions that have so far resisted existing therapies.

How is it though that we know certain microbes are associated with certain diseases? The easiest proof comes from a case where one specific microbe has a major impact on health, this describes over 100 years of research into infectious diseases. If you are exposed to a microbe such as Salmonella, you expect to get sick, and provided that you treat it with the right antibiotic you expect to get better. Hang on though; do you always get sick just because you have been exposed? The answer here is dependent on a combination of exposure, genetic makeup and other contributory factors. There are some people who are born with resistance to certain diseases. Where though does this resistance come from? It is this type of questioning that makes mice studies so popular amongst researchers. It is from these studies we have learnt susceptibility to every kind of infection hinges greatly on genetics.

We are beginning to realize that there may be many more diseases where we are all exposed to the same microbe, but it is dangerous to just a few of us, but more research is required at this time to figure out why.

The following is a roundup of the key diseases in which it is suspected that microbes play a part.

Inflammatory bowel disease

IBD, inflammatory bowel disease is a wide diagnosis for inflammation of the digestive tract. The really well known diseases that fall into this description are Crohn's disease and ulcerative colitis. These diseases have common characteristics which are that they have an altered relationship between the immune system and the intestinal microbes. In an attempt to target the pathogens which are infecting you, your body goes to war with all of the creatures in your intestines and the bleeding, intense pain and frequent trips to the toilet are all collateral damage.

One typical sign shared by these diseases is an increase in the number of certain bacteria. The most interesting thing is that the microbes in patients do not appear to be behaving in a normal way; this could be that their metabolism has been switched off and they are eating and secreting different chemicals. It is not yet known whether this altered behavior is caused by the body's immune response or whether it is the microbes that are at fault. Your immune system does not actually keep lists of good and bad microbe behavior. It is not clear yet whether these inflammatory bowel diseases are caused by a change in the microbiome or whether there is something in the genes of the afflicted that causes the body's normal relationship with gut microbes to go array and as such the changes in the microbial are just a response, maybe it is a combination of all of these factors.

Celiac disease is closely linked to IBD but also involves a component of the immune system as in eating wheat will see the natural gluten proteins in wheat activate the immune system, which attached the lining of the gut, shredding it. There has been vast interest into whether celiac is linked to microbiome however all studies have found that there are no consistent trends that associate microbes with celiac. Many studies are able to quantify the differences between the microbiome of celiac patients and healthy people and the bacteria in the celiac patients continue to be different. The links are still complex with far more work required to understand whether the bacteria in the stomach contributes to celiac or just respond to the altered gluten free diets.

Obesity

A gentleman and lady were struck down with a stomach bug, both recovered and it flared up again. They both took the same antibiotic and once they were on their feet again, they resumed the same diet and exercise regimes. The gentleman lost a vast amount of weight about 75lbs in a few months going from obese to a healthy weight. In contrast the lady lost no weight. Scientists believe that the difference was due to a radical change in the man's microbes. Both people responded differently to the same disease and were treated in the same way.

Although we cannot draw scientific conclusions from one study this story mirrors what a number of published studies are showing. We are continually learning that there is a strong microbial component to obesity. When normal sized germ free mice receive decal transplants from obese mice they get fatter. This experiment works regardless of whether the mouse was fat from being overfed an unhealthy diet or it was genetic mutation that made it fat.

You may wonder whether it is the microbes doing this or whether it is something else that is present in the stool. In order to answer this a team of researchers asked whether it would be possible to isolate hundreds of individual strains of bacteria from an individual person and grow each strain without the rest of the fecal matter, mix them together in similar proportions as in the original sample, then transfer the weight difference by transferring the bacteria to a new host. This is precisely what they did, so proving it was the microbes that were responsible for the weight gain, not a virus antibody, chemical or anything else in the stool.

However even more amazing is that by isolating bacteria from lean people, it would be possible to design a microbial community which prevented the mice from gaining weight which it would normally gain when housed with an obese mouse and exposed to its chubby microbes. Currently scientists have not been able to design a microbe community which will actually slim down the mouse or a person, but this is certainly their ongoing goal. There is unpublished research that reports using antibiotics to target the bacteria that grow on a high fat diet, have been successful at slimming the mouse even if it still eats an unhealthy diet.

There are many fad diets aimed at humans that target improving the person's microbiome; however there is very little evidence to substantiate whether these actually work. Currently there is not enough known about the ways in which certain microbes affect absorption and digestion in order to make any targeted intervention. Researchers at Harvard University published the results in 2011 which found that some foods are associated with weight gain and others weight loss. It will come as no surprise to learn that fat rich potato chips lead to weight gain, however the two foods most associated with weight loss are nuts and yoghurts even though both of these can be high in fat.

We know from studies in mice that specific microbes or combinations of microbes are associated with weight gain or loss. The question has to be could there be a connection between particular foods and the microbes that make us slimmer? There is a lot of evidence that proves what you eat alters your microbiome, making it more habitable for certain species and less for others. It has been proved by a professor of gastroenterology that a long tern diet of a year or more is linked very strongly with the overall microbiome. The team of researchers showed people that ate an abundance of carbohydrates tended to have a lot of Prevotella, whereas those who ate a lot of protein, particularly meat tended to have a lot of Bacteroides. These two types of bacteria help us to digest and metabolize our foods. It is yet to be proved what influence Bacteroides species have on typical weight related diseases such as diabetes and obesity but there are suggested links. It is really exciting to think we could grow ourselves healthier and leaner microbiome by simply changing our diets. There are some changes that can rapidly alter our microbes. Studies show that following a vegan diet showed little immediate change to the gut microbes, however following a meat and cheese diet caused huge changes overnight, increasing the types of bacteria that are linked to cardiovascular disease. Therefore an extreme diet has bad effects incredibly quickly yet the question is whether there is a diet that can provide good effects this fast.

Asthma and allergies

The idea that reduced microbial diversity leads to allergies and asthma dates back to the 80s where research showed later siblings in larger families tend to have lower rates of hay fever and related allergies. It was also suggested that catching infections from older siblings may help to train the immune system in order to target the real invaders. This practice is known as "hygiene hypothesis" which really suggests that keeping ourselves too clean can lead to problems in our immune system as by leaving our immune system idle and unchallenged by bacterial and viral pathogens leaves the system restless.

The focus has shifted away from the common infections such as colds, measles and flu which are now believed to be harmful. Instead the modern day hygiene hypothesis centers on our super clean childhoods, which keeps us protected from diverse microbes from healthy sources which range from soil to leaf, surfaces to domestic or wild animals. In order to understand this better imagine your immune system is a radio, if you are tuned to a particular station you can hear the music perfectly however if you are between stations random signals can lead to loud unpleasant static. If you are lucky it will be pollen or peanut butter that spikes through the static causing allergies however if you are unlucky the immune system may latch onto your own cells resulting in diabetes, multiple sclerosis or other autoimmune diseases.

The message here is for parents is that you still should not challenge your child's immune system by encouraging them to eat meat that is a few days old, lick the floor etc, or expose them to harmful bacteria but the modern hygiene hypothesis says that coming across good microbes from dirt, a wide range of people and animals may provide a good preventative medicine. The evidence for this is rapidly growing with Erika von Mutius from the children's hospital at the University of Munich being a pioneer in this area. She has shown that exposure to farming in early life substantially reduces the risk of asthma and allergies. Some of this effect can be explained by children coming in contact with straw, farm milk, cows as well as certain bacteria and fungi.

Some interesting findings suggest that microbial exposure when pregnant and not just childhood may be important for reducing allergic diseases. Promising yet preliminary results have shown that there are a number of probiotics that can relieve atopic disease and asthma and also that certain microbes can reverse allergies in mice and prevent or cause food allergies to develop.

The available data on whether breast milk can reduce the incidence of these diseases tend to show modest if any effects. Interestingly living in a setting with more varied microbes appears to decrease the risk of allergic disease. Being exposed prenatally and in the first year of life appears to decrease the risk of allergies later in life. Having dogs rather than children increased human microbial diversity for couples living together and exposure to dogs and cats during adolescence shows increases in the risk of eczema and asthma.

It is difficult to add up all of this evidence however recommendations could be summed up as follows:

Have a dog, ideally prenatally, live on a farm where your child or children are exposed to straw and cows, avoid antibiotics early in life and take probiotics. Generally exposure to diverse microbes seems to help even though scientists are still working out the specific microbes that are involved, and it could be that diversity is most important.

Kwashiorkor

Due to the world's struggle with its waistlines ingoing research is helping to provide a better understanding of the microbial component that is the cause of human suffering.

Kwashiorkor is a disease synonymous with distended bellies from the famine racked frames of those it afflicts. Kwashiorkor for a long time was thought of as a form of malnutrition occurring from a diet lacking in protein. This type of malnutrition is seen in countries where there are high levels of food insecurity and there is little access to nutritious affordable food. The obvious question is surely that the problem could be fixed by giving these people more food. However this is not always the case as providing more calories from rice and corn doesn't work. Providing a peanut butter based supplement fortified with vitamins, sugar and micronutrients has been proved to rescue about 80% of the malnourished children treated in famine stricken areas, but what about the other 20%? Why does the peanut but based supplement not work for them? The reason seems to be that kwashiorkor is not just a disease of malnutrition but also one of microbiome. Studies show that this peanut butter based supplement would help far more if it was combined with an initial dose of antibiotics to kill the bad microbes in the sick.

Ironically your microbiome can inflict stubborn obesity or persistent undernourishment. One can only hope that this knowledge will eventually help to solve the problems seen in both developed and underdeveloped countries alike.

There are some general trends emerging regarding links between diseases and microbiome. We have learnt that gut microbial communities with a lower diversity are associated with obesity, inflammatory bowel disease and rheumatoid arthritis. In microbial diversity there is strength, and we also seen that the type of bacteria that causes inflammation in the body are linked with health problems such as diarrhea, IBD and in some obesity.

Chapter 4 – How microbes affect your mind, mood and more

It is one thing to learn that the microbes present in your gut have a say in how well or sick you are or what your waistline looks like. However your mood, mind and behavior surely have nothing to do with microbes? As crazy as it may sound there is increasing evidence to show that our microbes do get a say in who we become and how we feel.

From their home in your stomach the microbes do not just influence the way you digest food, tolerate and absorb drugs, produce hormones and are capable of interacting with our immune systems which then affects our brains. Together the various interactions between microbes and our brain are called the microbiome – gut – brain – axis and being able to understand this axis may have profound implications for our understanding of psychiatric disorder and our nervous system. It has been proved that depression involves an inflammatory response and a number of beneficial bacteria in the gut produce short chain fatty acids such as butyrate which help feed the cells that line the gut to reduce the inflammation. Recently the microbiome has been linked to depression.

The ability of soil microbes to modulate the human immune system has led to many researchers suggesting it could be possible to make them into a vaccine against stress and depression. It has been suggested that our clean living could explain the rapid increase of diseases that involve inflammation such as diabetes, arthritis and depression.

With all of their influence on our body chemistry microbes may also be able to shape our minds as we develop and autism is a particularly interesting case. Studies have shown that children with autism spectrum disorders differ from neuro typical children in their gut microbiome. The idea that we are able to isolate the chemicals that are responsible for a particular condition even one that involves the brain and then be able to determine and identify the bacteria that either produce or eliminate these chemicals is particularly exciting.

Our microscopic passengers are also able to influence what we do and how we think, and sometimes it is our genes that determine which bacteria live within us, and then these bacteria turn around and influence how we behave. This point is extremely documented with an experiment where mice lacking a gene known as Tlr5 make them gorge and consume too much food becoming obese; this can be proved in two different experiments. In one experiment the Tlr5 less mice microbes are transferred into genetically normal mice who then overeat and become fat. In the other experiment antibiotics are used to wipe out the microbes in the Tlr5 less mice and their appetites then return to normal. It is amazing to think that a simple genetic tweak is capable of creating gut microbes which affect behavior and this behavior can then be transferred to another stomach and alter the original behavior of the host.

Appetite is not the only behavior influences by microbes, anxiety can also be effective. This can be seen when microbes are swapped between two genetically strains of mice as their performance in anxiety tests show. The microbiologist, Sven Pettersson saw higher anxiety amongst the mice raised in a bubble without any microbes, however if transferred the normal bacteria to mice within a few days of birth they will grow up to behave the same way as normal mice.

There are specific probiotics that have been shown to change behavior in both mice and humans and there are over 500 studies that link probiotics to behavior particularly depression and anxiety. The probiotic Lactobacillus helveticus can decrease the anxiety in mice and Lactobacillus reuteri can reduce the likelihood that mice will develop infections when they are stressed. Lactobacillus rhamnosus GG is reported to reduce obsessive compulsive behaviors and as we previously mentioned the probiotic strains of Bacteroides fragilis can save mice from some autistic style traits including repetitive behavior and cognitive deficits.

Although it is great to cure mice, there will come a time where you will want to also cure people and this is what biomedical science is pursuing. Certain probiotics have been used in clinical trials successfully and these include remedies for irritable bowel syndrome and early onset celiac disease. Both of these conditions are also frequently associated with depression. There are also reports that show using probiotics can alleviate the illness that is known as chronic fatigue syndrome. Healthy human volunteers undertook a study where they took Lactobacillus helvetic and Bifidobacterium longum after which they all reported improvements in their mood. Whilst this research is very much in the early stages the evidence for psychological effects of altering the microbiome and this is looking very promising. It is reported that a person who changes their diet can also change their mood and this could prove that changing your diet changing your microbes and it is therefore possible that some of these effects have a microbial component. If microbes can change our health and mind the question has to be can we change our microbes to improve ourselves?

Chapter 5 –Probiotics and how to build yourself better microbiome

Taking into consideration all that microbiomes can do for us we have to ask whether we can build ourselves a better one. We should be able to as we change our microbiomes all the time. If you change what you eat or the alcohol that you consume you are altering your microbiomes. You change it also if you use antimicrobial soap or are taking a prescribed course of antibiotics.

However, what if we did it purposefully? What would a microbe focused medicine look like? In order to understand this better think of your microbiome as the lawn in your garden. You start with a flourishing lawn with a little mix of flowers interspersed within the grass. In order to keep the grasses growing properly and remaining dominance you may want to fertilize it and this is where prebiotics take center stage.

Prebiotics

You may or may not have heard of prebiotics and to make it easier to understand you should think of prebiotics as fertilizer for your microbes providing nutrients required and which favor the beneficial species. Prebiotics are mainly soluble fibers such as lactulose, inulin, and glacto-oligosaccharides etc which are naturally found in a variety of fruits and vegetables. These ingredients are fermented by bacteria that live in the large intestine such as Ruminococcus gnavus. These produce short chain fatty acids like butyrate and these are what provide the nutrition for the cells that line the stomach.

Prebiotics are believed to reproduce a number of the benefits of a natural fiber rich diet by stimulating health promoting microbes. There is no single definition when it comes to prebiotics and in accordance with the International Scientific Association for Probiotics and Prebiotics they are defined as non digestible substances which provide a beneficial physiological effect for the host by selectively stimulating the favorable activity and or growth of a certain number of indigenous bacteria.

There have been some controlled clinical trials of prebiotics which showed they were beneficial in the treatment of constipation, Crohn's disease and insulin resistance however most of the clinical studies to date are still at the process of proving safety with the number of participants being too small to gain reliable conclusions about what they should do.

Probiotics

Let's go back to the earlier example of the lawn, currently it is lush and green then suddenly disaster strikes. Whether this is a flood or your grass is suddenly overrun with weeds, the question is what can you do? In this situation the time is right for you to reseed the lawn selectively.

Probiotics are mainly bacteria that are naturally found in the gut or in foods that have been fermented such as yogurt. Examples of probiotics are Bifidobacterium and Lactobacillus. Probiotics have a solid definition being live microorganisms that when taken in sufficient quantities benefit your health.

Also known as good bacteria or helpful bacteria, probiotics are available as dietary supplements, yogurt and suppositories. Some probiotic products contain just one strain of bacteria whereas others will contain a mixture of different types of bacteria and fungi. Currently there are no health claims that have been approved for probiotics and therefore they are currently marketed as food supplements.

There have been a number of clinical trials for probiotics with people becoming far more interesting in the past few years as they have got better at reading the microbiome. The majority of the strongest evidence supports the therapeutic and preventive effects that probiotics have had on children and suffering from diarrhea and adults who have the symptoms of irritable bowel syndrome. Promising results that have been shown with the use of probiotics include the prevention and reduction of a severe intestinal condition of premature newborns that is known as necrotizing enterocolitis. Future applications include using probiotics to treat obesity, reducing cholesterol and managing irritable bowel syndrome. There are a wide variety of possible effects from probiotics which include the production of antimicrobial compounds and keeping harmful bacteria at bay by competing for nutrients and prebiotics.

Surprisingly the probiotics do not need to survive to have an effect; sometimes they can alter your gut bacteria behavior by just passing through. The main problem with probiotics is that there is far more hype that there is actual solid research.

Have you looked at probiotics in your supermarket recently? There are a number of supermarkets that now dedicate an entire wall to microbes that are supposed to improve the health of your gut. However any actual evidence to support these claims is still lacking. The principles that have led to the isolation of certain microbes are sound but the majority has not been proved to work for these conditions. It is also still debatable whether the preparations offered for sale contain any living organisms after all they have been shipped then sat on the shelf in the supermarket and we know that these micro organisms require very specific conditions to survive.

The biggest problem however is that many people assume that any probiotic will do the job, however this is not an assumption we would make for any other product. Imagine telling a friend that you were not feeling well and you had heard of a drug that could help, so you took it and felt better. One thing is certain, and this is that they are likely to question your actions, for example which drug your took and why you took a certain drug rather than another. Alternatively they could ask whether there is any solid evidence that the drug works for the medical condition you have and what street corner you had brought said drug from!

These questions are very rarely asked about probiotics. I recently had a similar conversation with a friend who had tried a couple of probiotics which had failed to treat her irritable bowel symptoms that had flared up after a large dose of antibiotics. I asked how she had chosen the probiotics she had tried and she said that one had been recommended by a friend and the other by the pharmacist. I suggested that she tried one that had randomized, controlled trial data that suggests it would work for IBS. She did complain about how much more expensive this was, however the following day she reported that the probiotic worked brilliantly, far better than anything else she had tried. Now after almost a year she has her IBS under control seemingly due to the probiotic that she has been taking.

Whilst this is just one example, it reinforces the idea that when it comes to anything medical, science can be most helpful. Therefore it is worth asking your pharmacist for a probiotic that has controlled trials to back them up. Failing this, live yogurt is unlikely to hurt and has helped a huge number of people. However the limited clinical data that is available suggests even different kinds of live yogurt differ substantially in how much they can help.

Fecal transplants

Back to the lawn example used previously, there will be times where you have no option but to tear up your whole lawn and then lay down fresh turf.

People that suffer with severe gastrointestinal illness really can poop themselves to death. Those who suffer with a disease such as Clostridium difficile associated diarrhea have to visited the bathroom dozens of times a day and this disease is often life threatening as well as being one of the biggest infections contracted in hospital, infecting over 300,000 people and killing about 15,000 a year.

Many people take antibiotics to treat C diff however they often fail. To complement or replace the antibiotics the patients may be given microbes from someone who is healthy. One such experimental treatment for C diff is fecal transplantation. This is exactly as it sounds and is where a healthy relative donates a stool sample which is then diluted and given to the patient. There are two ways in which these transplants can take place and both are effective in 90% of those suffering from C diff.

Research undertaken at the University of Minnesota showed C diff patients have stool communities that bear no resemblance to those of a healthy adult and their fecal microbes are similar to those in the skin or vagina. Within a few days of fecal transplantation their gut communities are restored to normal and their symptoms have completely disappeared. Fecal transplantation is able to restore the complete ecosystem in the gut. Currently this procedure has only been used for dire cases of C diff however its success has been astounding and researchers are keen to discover what other conditions this could help.

Vaccines

Continuing further with the lawn example, what if you could stop your lawn from getting sick in the first place?

Vaccination is one of the most effective public health treatments we know of with vaccines proving to be over 90% effective against the diseases that they can treat and have saved more lives all over the world than any innovation with the exception of clean water.

Vaccines are the greatest triumph that human's have produced in public health. Typically, they only need to be taken a few times in childhood to provide positive protection and preventing illnesses from ever occurring over a lifetime. Smallpox is a disease that has been known of since the time of the pharaoh's and has been responsible for killing millions of people and blinding millions more; however thanks to vaccinations the disease has been eradicated.

Vaccines are very specific and train the immune system to respond to particular bacteria which is often a species or individual strain and not targeting the good bacteria. To date vaccines have primarily be used for individual pathogens, beginning with the nastiest. As the list of vaccines expand less severe kinds of microbes are being targeted, including those that may kill you years after they have infected you rather than immediately.

Given with what is being discovered about the role of particular types of bacteria in various diseases that have not been vaccinated against, surely we could start to vaccinate against them? For example, would it be possible for a vaccine to be developed against the bacteria which produces a chemical known as trimethylamine – N – oxide which leads to cardiovascular problems or against Fusobacterium nucleatum which is found in tumors in colon cancer, or even against types of gut bacteria that efficiently help us to extract energy from an unhealthy diet and from becoming obese? Currently these are simply questions; however the potential for the future is vast.

How about vaccinating against post traumatic stress disorder or depression? The World Health Organization has reported that depression is the leading cause of disability in America and is rapidly becoming more common worldwide. The increases in the rate of depression match the rise of other diseases such as inflammatory bowel disease, diabetes and multiple sclerosis which have both immune and microbial components. Could our soil bacteria which modulate the immune system play a role?

Experiments have been undertaken on mice and a soil bacterium that is known as Mycobacterium vaccae and shown to reduce anxiety. Surprisingly a social stress situation M. vaccae treatment shows that the mice are far more resilient against the effects from stress possibly providing a base for treating stress disorders in humans.

Chapter 6 – The future of human microbiome

The previous chapters of this book should have provided you with far more knowledge and an understanding of human microbiome. The rate of progress in microbial science is amazing as the discoveries that are being made are revelations that promise in every step to reshape and deepen our understanding of the basic ways our bodies and minds work.

In just a few years we have gone from understanding that our microbial cells outnumber our human cells to discovering that their genes outnumber ours even further, and understanding that microbes may shortly be able to explain all manner of health and sickness that until now have been a mystery. It has only been in the last few years that it has been cheap enough for us to place our own personal mark in the microbial map, and to see how this relates to other people. It is a thrilling time to be studying microbes and taking your own swabs is a small price to pay as we move forwards.

The newly discovered microbial frontier now extends even further than our bodies as we are beginning to learn how microbes everywhere relate to one another. The technology that allows us to read the human microbiome can also be applied to our pets, wild animals, livestock and even the planet itself. With all of our new found knowledge, microbes can be viewed as a web that connects the health of humans, animals and the environment and we may eventually understand how to improve the microscopic ecosystems that we live in and those that live within us.

Some of the most exciting breakthroughs to come include the following:

- Tests that are based on your microbes that can tell how you will respond to painkillers, heart drugs and artificial sweeteners
- Better understanding of how your body including its microbes response to diet and exercise and what you should personally do to become healthier
- Thorough understanding of stool transplants and whether everybody's poop is equally curative or whether a donor match is needed. We also being to question whether a poop pill could be used instead

In the future the following proactive questions are to be vigorously pursued:

1. Is it possible to design microbial communities that can protect humans from weight gain in the same way that works for mice?
2. Will it be possible to design microbes that can live on our skin and repel mosquitoes?
3. Can microbes be used not only to diagnose but also to cure the vast array of diseases that we now know they have involvement with?

There is still a long way to go on our journey of microbial discovery. Currently we are extremely good at finding which microbes flourish in particular environments, however we currently do not yet know what the microbes are doing or how they talk to each other or us. We also have no idea what the unintended consequences of disturbing the microbes are and whether using antibiotics to kill bad bugs or introducing new types of microbes via our diets, our interaction with other people and animals or our contact with the environment are all ways forward.

One of the biggest parts of the challenge right now is that our microbiomes are changing every day, and we are doing this in an undirected manner. The true power of microbiome science will be unveiled when we really understand what we need to do in order to achieve a desired effect on the complete ecosystem within us.

In order to start building this system, hundreds of scientists have got together and become involved in the Human Microbiome Project, the Earth Microbiome Project and the American gut. These scientists along with thousands of members of the public providing samples and support have made these projects possible. The Human Microbiome Project has been created to gather a genetic census of a healthy microbiome and the changes from it in a variety of diseases. American gut aims to broaden that census and include a greater variation of sick and healthy people. The Earth Microbiome Project plans to look further than humans to microbial communities in our planet's ecosystems.

All three of the projects are ground breaking, primed to expand our capability to go from description to prescription. The research to come will eventually provide us with not only detailed microbial maps of humanity but also a kind of guiding body of knowledge that will tell us not only where we are but also where we want to go and how we can go about getting there.

Conclusion

I want to thank you for choosing to read "What's going on in your gut? - The complete guide to Probiotics, and the health benefits they offer." I hope that you have found the information interesting and easy to relate to your life.

The work that I have highlighted in this book involves a vast and ever growing research community that includes scientists, volunteers and those we must not forget, the mice!

There are vast numbers of microbes in our bodies and our homes, many of these are good for us but there are some that are bad. As our knowledge of the microbes and germs that populate our living space become apparent the easier it will be to have an environment that encourages happy and healthy microbes.

Once again thank you for taking the time to read this book and you now have the knowledge required to move further towards living with your own healthy microbes.

-- Martin Meyer

Did you enjoy this book?

I want to thank you for purchasing and reading this book. I really hope you got a lot out of it.

Can I ask a quick favor though?

If you enjoyed this book I would really appreciate it if you could leave me a positive review on Amazon.

I love getting feedback from my customers and reviews on Amazon really do make a difference. I read all my reviews and would really appreciate your thoughts.

Thanks so much.

Martin Meyer.